Oh!

It's Just You,

Cancer

BISHOP EARL P. PAULK

Printed in the United States of America
ISBN 0-917595-59-9

About the Title

The title of this book came from a very interesting source—a message preached at the Cathedral several years ago by Bishop Donnie Meares.[1] He told the congregation that evil spirits had often manifested themselves in unusual ways to torment him. He described how demonic forces had attacked him during the night, shaking the clothes in his closet and causing them to sway back and forth, as though moved by unseen hands. One night an unusual sound awakened him. The Bishop sat up in his bed, startled. Once again, he sensed the presence of an evil force in his bedroom. Tired of his torment, he laid back down, turned over and said, "Oh, it's just you, Devil." With that, he went back to sleep.

When we hear the word "cancer," we are frequently filled with dread, even outright fear. We shun the use of the word, preferring to call it the "Big C" or some other less intimidating name. Why? Because cancer usually means a terrible struggle—maybe even death—for us or for someone we love. I have come to believe that we must reach a place of confidence when dealing with cancer and overcome the fear associated with its diagnosis. We need the kind of confident faith we see in the story told by Bishop Meares. I believe that it is time for us to rise in faith and boldly say to our tormentor, *"Oh! It's just you, cancer"* and then get back to the real business of the Kingdom of God.

---

[1] Bishop Donnie Meares *is the senior pastor of Evangel Cathedral in Washington, D.C., and a bishop over many churches in several countries.*

Dedication

This book is dedicated to one of the most unique women I have ever met, Alma Blackmon. She has fought and won the battle with cancer more than once over the years. Alma spends much of her time giving hope to other cancer patients. She sends out monthly letters of encouragement. When Alma found out that I had cancer, she immediately put me on her prayer list, along with the others who are a part of her ministry for cancer patients, and started to send me helpful books and information. A woman of many talents and tremendous commitment, Alma has taught some of the most outstanding musicians of our day, including members of Take Six and Wintley Phipps. Not only did she teach, but she also raised Brenda Wood, one of the outstanding news anchors in the nation and the face of one of Atlanta's leading television stations. An unfailing encouragement in times of need, with an intuitive sense that always knows just when to call, Alma Blackmon has turned her personal struggle into more than a personal triumph. She is a source of hope for many—including myself. With great joy and heart-felt gratitude for her friendship, I dedicate this book to her.

Special Thanks

When compiling a book it takes many people to make it successful. First of all I would like to thank Zully Hunter for her thorough research on the subject of cancer and for writing much of this book. She spent countless hours pouring over my own personal notes and sermons as well as made numerous phone calls to outstanding physicians aroud the world in order to obtain helpful materials about cancer and advancements in curing this dreaded disease.

I would also like to thank Pastor Chad Hyatt for unselfishly giving his time to writing and editing this work. Without his support, this book would not have become a reality.

Special thanks to Wendy Long for her assistance to Pastor Chad Hyatt, Charlotte Lemons for layout and to LaDonna Diaz, Jill Lancaster, and Libby Pratt for proofreading.

Whatever good may be accomplished by this work, much of the credit should go to this staff, but we desire that all glory should be given to God.

Acknowledgements

I want to give God the glory for my healing and for walking with me throughout many gloomy days of cancer treatment and its painful side effects. I thank Him for being faithful to His promises and for sending His Word of healing.

To my dear wife, Norma, I express both my appreciation and my love for being with me every step of the way during my battle against cancer. Thank you for your unconditional love for me.

To my family and to those I consider part of my family, thank you for your constant support and love toward me.

To my outstanding pastoral staff and to the wonderful congregation at the Cathedral of the Holy Spirit, thank you for your faith, love, and prayers for me.

To my dear friend, Tommy Reid, a special man of God, thank you for being obedient to the Lord and speaking His heart at the appointed time.

To Benny Hinn, I want to express my great appreciation for going out of your way to come to the Cathedral to pray for me and for those in my congregation who needed to receive their healing.

To my beloved friend, Alma Blackmon, thank you for never ceasing to encourage me and to send me vital information on cancer.

To Dr. Guishan Harjee, Dr. Thomas Schoborg, Dr. Hamilton Williams and Dr. Michael Goodman, whose knowledge, skills, and expertise assisted me in my fight against cancer, thank you.

And finally, I want to thank everyone here in the United States and all over the world that prayed for me and sent me a word of encouragement. May God richly bless you.

Earl Paulk

Introduction

Not long ago, God spoke to my spirit and told me that my church, the Cathedral of the Holy Spirit, would become a spiritual healing center for cancer. Shortly after I shared this with my congregation, several members of our church were diagnosed with cancer, including myself. Though we do not like to hear it, a great personal price must often be paid to become all that God has promised us we'll be.

In my own life, I have gone through many battles which, though very painful and difficult, have always resulted in a deepening of the work of God's grace in me. I know through personal experience what it is to be depressed and to be afflicted with illness. Like many of you, I have lost loved ones, including my parents, my baby sister, and my oldest daughter. I have seen the smoldering remains of my home after it was destroyed by fire, taking with it personal writings and decades of study notes, family heirlooms, and personal photographs that can never be replaced. Yet through all of this, I have strived to stay on track spiritually, emotionally, and physically. I have always tried to keep a healthy body through regular exercise and eating right. None of that fully prepared me for what took place in the Fall of 1999. Sitting in my doctor's office, I heard him say words that seemed unbelievable to me: "You have prostate cancer." My first struggle came immediately. I found it difficult to imagine that there could be a way through what then seemed like the end of the road. Later, I realized God had already gone before me.

More than a year prior to being diagnosed with cancer, my good friend of many years, Pastor Tommy Reid[1], gave me a word of prophecy. This promise helped carry me through my journey with cancer. While it is lengthy, I give it to you in its entirety just as he spoke it during a Sunday morning service at the Cathedral. Perhaps you too will find strength in its promises. He said:

> *"God shall extend your years as you begin to move more and more in the dimension of eternal presence. That will affect even the natural aging process of your body. You could easily be a fifty or sixty-year-old man at ninety, because God does not*

measure our life in years, but in fulfilled purpose. Your purpose, sir, is far from being fulfilled or finished. You have much of the race yet to be run. Your prophetic voice has yet to be apprehended by the world. You will come to know, as you have never known, the dimension of Matthew, Chapter Ten. You will soon discover, as you have never discovered, the hours, the powers of the age to come, invading this present age. Remember Abraham and Sarah, young at a hundred. Remember Moses beginning his career at eighty. So shall your years be—not just long in years but, sir, long in youth. You shall stand strong and straight and powerful many more years. For you shall drink of that living water. You shall taste of the powers of the age to come, and when you drink them, it will give you life.

You have known in your life the sorrows of premature deaths of those you dearly loved. But you will now enter a new dimension of the powers of the age to come, a power of which you have only dreamed. There will come a day when again you will stand face to face with death, but this time, as you live more and more in the powers of the age to come, you shall rob death of its prey. Life shall replace death. You are to remember the graphic example I have shown you in this ministry. Satan declared death to this house. Many other great houses that were built by your contemporaries have succumbed to Satan's decree of death. But you defied death, and you replaced it with life. Your prophetic voice replaced death in this place with life. Look around you and see the life—a demonstration of the living power of the age to come. You are to stand tall.

You now play tennis with great strength at seventy. You shall play with as great a strength at ninety. You know that now you preach with greater strength and anointing than you did at fifty. Your voice will not fade, nor your back bend, nor your eyes dim, nor your mind lack clarity, for you shall know the power of the age to come. You will taste it. Its waters will be sweet to your taste, and fill even your

*physical body with its life. Drink from
that water. It is the sweetest water that
has ever been birthed."*

During my battle against cancer, I discovered
anew that our spirituality and our physical health
are deeply connected. God is very much concerned
about our health. Through our healthy, long lives,
He proves the benefits of keeping His covenant and
helps us to fulfill our own individual purpose. Make
no mistake about it, we did not come into this world
by accident but by God's will. He has given each of
us a unique destiny—a God-given assignment—to
fulfill. And He watches over our lives with great
care to help us accomplish that assignment. More-
over, God is a loving Father who is moved with compassion toward His children, and He wants us to
have an abundant life. Through His love and care,
God has given us both spiritual and natural guidelines to follow in order to keep our bodies in good
health and to restore them to that health when they
become sick.

Most of all, however, I have learned how my
own experience could help others. My calling as a
pastor does not insulate me from the troubles of life.
I have discovered that when I respond to my own

challenges with faith, they become redemptive experiences that can bring comfort to others. My goal in this little book is to share with you my experience and the way that God cares for us so that you too will be able to find comfort and practical answers in your time of trouble. In these pages, you will find truth and encouragement, in addition to good medical information. In my time of weakness, I found a relationship with God greater than I had ever known and a well of spiritual strength more powerful than I had ever experienced. In the midst of my infirmity, I was able to stand up and give God the glory.

[1]Tommy Reid *is the senior pastor at Full Gospel Tabernacle in Buffalo, New York*

Contents

ONE

Releasing the Virtue That is in Jesus

Jesus Came to Bring Abundant Life

When Jesus began His ministry, He declared that the words of the prophet Isaiah were fulfilled in Him: *"The Spirit of the Lord is upon Me, because He has anointed Me to preach the gospel to the poor. He has sent Me to heal the brokenhearted, to preach deliverance to the captives and recovery of sight to the blind, to set at liberty those who are oppressed, to preach the acceptable year of the Lord"* (Luke 4:18-19). This prophetic quotation was a kind of "platform" statement for His evangelistic mission. From that moment on, there was no doubt as to what Jesus was here to do. He made it clear that He was here to bring life and to set us free from those things that bind us.

Sometimes in presenting Jesus, we preachers forget the part of His ministry that brought healing to people. An example of how central healing was to His overall ministry can be found in Matthew 9:35-38, which is the foundational scripture for our ministry at the Cathedral of the Holy Spirit. Earlier in the chapter, Matthew tells us that

> *"When Jesus departed from there, two blind men followed Him crying out, saying, 'Son of David, have mercy on us.' And when He had come into the house, the blind men came to Him, and Jesus said to them, 'Do you believe that I am able to do this?' And they said, 'Yes, Lord!' Then He touched their eyes and said, 'According to your faith, be it unto you,' and their eyes were opened."* (Matt. 9:27-30).

Then Matthew records:

> *"Jesus went about all over the cities and villages teaching in their synagogues, preaching the gospel of the Kingdom, and healing every sickness*

*and every disease among the people. But when
He saw the multitudes, He was moved with compassion for them, because they were weary and
scattered, like sheep having no shepherd. Then
He said to His disciples, 'The harvest truly is plen-
tiful, but the laborers are few. Therefore, pray
the Lord of the harvest to send laborers into the
harvest.'"* (Matt. 9:35-38)

If we are a Christian church, and we are following the Head of the church, Jesus Christ, then we
have an obligation to be concerned for the healing
of the sick.

Resources for Healing

God continually provides resources for our well-
being in every area of life. He has made available
many resources to protect our health and to help us
to recover from illness. We have physical resources,
such as the immune system, nutrition, prevention,
and medical care. We have psychological resources
like positive thinking, self-encouragement, meditation, and emotional support. And we have spiritual resources: prayer, fasting, the Lord's Supper,

worship, and a covenant community of love.[1] Many people are familiar with the provisions of medical science, but few are aware of the other resources that God has given us. Above all else, we have faith in Jesus Christ. There is no more powerful resource during difficult times.

We must never forget that the gospel of the Kingdom as preached by Jesus is a message of hope because of God's grace—not despair because of sin. In fact, why we became sick isn't even the issue. Sickness has simply created an opportunity for God's redemptive work to be seen in our lives. Sickness, when faced with faith, regardless of its cause, will bring us closer to our Creator. He knows our frame—both our strengths and our weaknesses. The cross tells us that our Healer suffered just as we do and that by His wounds we are healed. Even if your life has been lived in rebellion against God, and you feel the things you suffer now are the consequences of things you have done in the past, there is *always* hope when you turn your life over to God. He never rejects us. And we simply cannot afford to reject the very source of our own healing. As the writer of Hebrews compassionately reminds us, *"He Himself said, 'I will never leave you nor forsake you'"*

(13:5)..Listen to the words of the One who created you:

> *"But now, thus says the Lord,*
> *Who created you, O Jacob,*
> *And He who formed you, O Israel:*
> *Fear not, for I have redeemed you;*
> *I have called you by your name;*
> *You are Mine.*
> *When you pass through the waters,*
> *I will be with you;*
> *And through the rivers,*
> *They shall not overflow you.*
> *When you walk through the fire,*
> *You shall not be burned.*
> *Nor shall the flame scorch you.*
> *For I am the Lord your God,*
> *The Holy One of Israel, your Savior..."*
> Isaiah 43:1-3

Your Relationship With Jesus Promotes Healing

When we accept Jesus as our Savior, all of God's promises become ours. God's strength and power are ours, and our possibilities are endless. Because of our new relationship with Jesus, we have the bold confidence of a son or daughter before God. We are entitled to all that He has promised us because we are His children. This confidence, this blessed assurance, gives our hearts a deep and abiding peace that works to promote healing. Fear, as we know, is a powerful emotion that often inhibits the immune system and slows down healing. As our relationship with God grows, faith takes the place of fear. We are set free from the fear of death. We begin to live in the reality that nothing is impossible with God—or for those who put their trust in Him.

Jesus came for two important reasons. He came, first of all, to give life and to give it abundantly. Abundant life means health and prosperity. It means a reason to live beyond our own narrow self-interest. Second, Jesus also came to destroy what the Bible calls the "works of the devil" (I John 3:8). If you had any doubt about it, know for sure that sickness and poverty are the works of the devil. Jesus shows us the character of God. He shows us that God's love has the power to heal us, spiritually and physically. By revealing the love and compassion of our Heavenly Father, Jesus accomplished His mission—both to give life and to destroy those things that bring death.

Whenever we feel unworthy to be healed, or even to live, we must remember what Jesus did for us. The Bible tells us that He became sin on the cross so that we might become righteous through Him (2 Cor. 5:21). Jesus was without sin, but He chose to take our sin upon Himself because of His great love for us. On the other hand, we're not righteous, but we become righteous through Jesus. Notice the exchange: His righteousness for our sin. This grace comes into our lives through faith. Our faith in Jesus means that we can stand before God with complete confidence—not because we've done anything deserving of His favor, but because of what Jesus has done for us. When we pray, instead of saying, "God, I am not worthy of you healing me," we can now say: "In the name of Jesus Christ who is righteous, I claim the healing of my body, because He became my sin." Passages like 1 Peter 2:24 remind us that Jesus took both our infirmities and our sins: *"who Himself bore our sins in His own body on the tree, that we, having died to sins, might live for righteousness— by whose stripes you were healed."*

Jesus: The Enemy of Sickness

See Jesus for who He is. He is the enemy of your sickness. If He came to destroy the works of Satan, then He came to destroy the disease that seeks your life. Jesus has set us free, not only from sin, but from all the powers of darkness—so that we can enjoy abundant life. No matter what kind of sickness you have, it is your enemy. But remember: Christ in you is greater than the sickness in you. His power is stronger than any disease that has declared war on your life. Listen to the confident boast of the psalmist; it's our declaration of victory, too:

"The Lord is my light and my salvation;
Whom shall I fear?
The Lord is the strength of my life;
Of whom shall I be afraid?
When the wicked came against me
To eat up my flesh,
My enemies and foes,
They stumbled and fell.
Though an army should encamp against me,
My heart shall not fear;
Though war should rise against me,
In this I will be confident."
Psalm 27:1-3

Jesus: The Door to Salvation, Healing, and Deliverance

Even though there are powerful forces that want to destroy our life, Jesus is on our side. Think of Jesus as God's door to salvation, healing, and deliverance. If the forces of hell have a strangle-hold on your life, knock on that door. Deliverance is on the other side. And don't give up knocking. Knock until you see it open. More often than not, persistence is the missing key to our victory. When we surrender everything to Jesus, the forces of darkness no longer have control over our lives. The power of God is released in us as we become open to God.

The Jesus who frees us deserves our praise. So take a moment now. Don't focus on the disease. Focus on Jesus. Open yourself to God, and let praise come out of your mouth. Praise is simply telling God who He is. He's the Creator who knows you and cares for you. He's the Healer who shares your suffering. He's the Door to abundant life. It doesn't really matter what the problem or need may be, just that Jesus represents the solution for it. The more we praise Jesus and lift Him up, the more we receive the abundance of life. Take advantage of the prayers and scriptures given at the end of this book for your encouragement.

Praise God in the middle of your trouble. And you will find God in the middle of your trouble. It's not that praise or faith makes God suddenly take notice of you. Truth is, He's been beside you all along. Praise and faith just help us to take notice of God. They help us to see the One who has been there with us, even when we felt abandoned. And they open us to God's possibilities in the middle of our impossibilities.

---

[1] Daniel E. Fountain, M.D.,*God, Medicine and Miracles* (Illinois, Harold Shaw Publisher, 1999).

TWO

The Kingdom of God and Healing

Divine Health

Growing up in a Pentecostal family, I believed in what we called "divine healing." We were committed to the doctrine that God had provided healing for believers through the atonement of Christ (that is, through the redemptive death and suffering of Jesus on the cross). Of course, we knew that medicine and physicians were there to aid us in case we had to call on them for help. But believing in divine healing meant that our first responsibility was to trust God for the healing of our bodies. Yet, with all the emphasis on divine healing, not a lot was said about divine *health*. Recently, however, God began to impress upon me more about the idea of divine health—that God not only heals us when we become sick but also wants us to embrace a healthy lifestyle that can prevent sickness.

Power and Authority

Jesus began His own ministry as a healing Messiah. Eventually, He commissioned twelve disciples to spread His ministry by preaching the gospel of the Kingdom. But He told them to do more than just preach. Jesus also made sure that He gave them authority over demons and the power to heal sickness. It is significant that Jesus gave them both power and authority. There is a difference between the two. Power is something that can be displayed, but authority is something that is resident in the person to whom it has been given. Later, Jesus sent seventy other disciples, telling them, *"Whatever city you enter, and they receive you, eat such things as are set before you. And heal the sick who are there, and say to them, 'The Kingdom of God has come near to you'"* (Luke 10:8-9). Jesus put both a resident authority and a demonstrative power within the disciples whom He sent out to heal, just as He himself had led a ministry in which healing was a vital ingredient.

The Kingdom of God and Healing

If we observe the practice of Jesus, clearly there is no separation between healing and the Kingdom of God or between preaching the gospel and casting out devils. All too often, however, we have interpreted healing in the church as *only* sponsoring hospitals and doing things that provide medical help to people. I am very grateful for such activities of the church, because they are, without doubt, an extension of God's cause. But I do not believe hospitals were what Jesus had in mind when He commissioned the disciples.

When Jesus had finished His ministry, He was crucified. After His ascension, God poured out the Holy Spirit on His disciples. The Acts of the Apostles records the very first thing that the disciples did after this outpouring. When Peter and John went up to the temple, a man, whom the Bible describes as "lame from his mother's womb," asked them for alms. Peter replied, *"Silver and gold I do not have, but what I do have I give to you; In the name of Jesus Christ of Nazareth, rise up and walk"* (Acts 3:6). The first example after Pentecost of the Holy Spirit moving through the early church was the healing of this lame man. It doesn't take much of a look around the church today to recognize that, somewhere along the way, we've lost something.

Jesus Gave His Church the Power and Authority to Heal

When Jesus gave authority to His disciples, He said that His followers—the church—should heal others. One of the reasons that we have been reluctant to recognize the full implications of Jesus' commission is because we often focus on the personality of the healer instead of looking at the power in the name of Jesus. I consider this attitude to be one of the greatest hindrances to healing in the Body of Christ today. Jesus went to the cross and delivered us from our sins. Both our sins and our diseases, which have been a curse upon humanity, were nailed to the cross. It's not the name of a person with a great healing ministry that saves and heals us. We are made whole by the name of Jesus and through the power of the Holy Spirit. I believe that when we come into the presence of God for worship, we ought to anticipate something happening in our bodies as well as within spirits. The most effective healing ministers today seem to recognize this. They seek to bring a congregation into the presence of God through prayer and the ministry of music before beginning to pray for the sick.

It Is Finished

When Judas betrayed Jesus, Jesus did not challenge him. Instead, He said, "This is your hour." The time belonged to the power of darkness (Luke 22:53). It was the hour of Satan, sickness, and rebellion. In fact, when Jesus was on the cross, He said, "It is finished" (John 19:30). Immediately, darkness came over the earth, filling the entire atmosphere. But the darkness did not last. On the third day, Jesus came out of the darkness of the tomb at the breaking of day. And from *that* hour, the power of darkness no longer prevailed. The power of darkness is no longer in charge of the universe, because Jesus Christ, the risen Lord, has put down the power of the enemy through his passion and resurrection.

Satan refuses to recognize this. In fact, he acts as if he was still in charge. But Jesus said that Satan no longer has power and authority over us. Paul declared, *"Having disarmed principalities and powers,*

He made a public spectacle of them, triumphing over them in [the cross]" (Col. 2:15). Satan is defeated. When you resist the devil, he will flee from you. It is our responsibility, therefore, not to allow him to invade our lives. As children of God, and by virtue of the blood of Jesus, we have the authority to drive the devil out of our lives. Anything that brings death or disqualifies us is not the plan of God. It's just another attack from an already defeated enemy.

As long as we fail to understand that the devil no longer has power over humanity, he will continue to come into the areas of our life that we leave open to him. Trust me, he won't just walk away and give up. He continually attacks us, trying to make us believe that he is still in charge. But since the resurrection, Satan is nothing more than a trespasser. The earth is the Lord's—not the devil's. Jesus said that the Kingdom of God has already come near when we are healed by the power of God. The Kingdom of God is not on hold. God's rule is already here and present with us. God isn't waiting to ascend to the throne; He's already there!

Where the work of the enemy is seen through the evidence of sickness and disease, we can now also see the evidence of God's Kingdom. It's what

Paul called "righteousness and peace and joy" in the Holy Spirit (Rom 14:17). Where sorrow and death once reigned as kings, now God's healing power and the joy of victory can be found. And again, our praise—the recognition of who God is— is critical for our experience of the Kingdom. When we praise Him, the Kingdom of God—with all of its blessings—has come near us. But when we fail to give God the glory He deserves—the glory owed a king—we put an enemy, who has already been deposed, back on the throne of our lives.

Steps to Divine Health:

1. *Remember that you were created to be whole.* You were not created to spend your life in disease and sickness. That's not God's original plan. It's the work of an enemy in your life. There was no sickness in the Garden of Eden. Adam and Eve ate the produce of the earth. They lived in a healthy environment. The garden is a prototype of God's intention for you. God wants to make us an example of His presence to such degree that wherever we are people will see the wholeness of Christ.

2. *Keep in mind that the powers of darkness had their hour until Jesus dethroned them.* Jesus came to destroy the works of the devil. Don't forget that the cross of Christ has defeated the powers that bring darkness into our world. Remind the devil of his defeat. We live in victory over the forces of disease and discouragement by the power of the Holy Spirit. Resist the devil, the Bible says, and he will flee. One way to resist the devil is not making a place for him.

3. *Be cheerful and joyful in the Holy Spirit.* Jesus commanded us to be of good cheer. That has to do with our attitude. God has always been concerned about your health. He has already given you a plan of recovery. God *wants* to make you whole. He is already at work in your life. So rejoice! We may weep for a time, but God does not want you to be overcome by sorrow. Don't think about the sorrow of the past but the exciting things that are about to take place in the future. Proverbs says, "A merry heart does good like medicine, but a broken spirit dries the bones" (17:22).

4. *Realize that God has built health into the universe, but you have to seek it.* God's King-dom—His rule, His order—is in every cell of your body. The potential for health is in ev-ery system, placed there by God. We see this in the way the body works to heal itself from injury and illness. God made it that way. The worst diseases, in fact, are often a perversion of that principle. Do the things that help your body heal itself.

5. *Understand that there is no such thing as hopelessness for the Christian.* The power of healing is in our sense of hope. Hope is what keeps you from giving up, even on bad days. Keep in mind that there is something greater than what you are experiencing to-day. Never count God out.

Total Health for the Total Person

Paul said that we should be sanctified com-pletely: in spirit, soul, and body (I Thes.23). The part of us that the Bible calls spirit is the part of us that is able to commune with God. The soul can be described as our self-awareness. And the body is like the living house where we reside. All of these—the spirit, the soul, and the body—form what I call the total person. Our care for the total person—not just one aspect of it—is critical to our overall health.

Whether we like it or not, we're at war for our health. We must be on guard against the enemies of the total person. The enemies of your spirit are numerous. Rebellion against God, procrastination in pursuit of your calling, inhibition in praise, and failure to prioritize are just a few. Defend your soul against foes like anxiety, depression, hopelessness, and feelings of unworthiness. Your body also has its enemies. We should avoid unnecessary stress, extremes in diet and exercise, and excess in eating and drinking. It's time to fight for our total health.

Some Ingredients for Total Health:

1. *Learn how to fight disease and sickness.* Fight it—with medicine and faith. Make up your mind to fight anything opposed to your quality of life by any means necessary.

2. *Say in your heart, "I know that I can be healed."* The leper said to Jesus, "If you will, you can heal me" (Luke 17:12-14). He knew Jesus could. But Jesus said, "I will." The woman that lay on her bed bleeding reached the point where she said, "If I can touch Jesus, I know I will be made whole" (Matt. 9:20-21). We must learn to say not only that God can heal, but that He will.

3. *Learn how to cry out for help.* Don't sit silently in your problems. Bartimaeus was a blind man, who sat by the side of the road and begged (Matt. 10:46-52). When he heard that Jesus was passing his way, he started crying out. "Jesus!" he shouted. The crowd admonished him to keep quiet. But that didn't stop Bartimaeus. He yelled even louder. When Jesus came over to him, the blind man explained, "I just want to see, Jesus—oh, that I might see!" Jesus responded, "Let it be to you according to your faith." If you yell long enough, you'll get someone's attention. Don't give up. Just keep crying out. Your cry for help can turn into faith.

4. ***Don't give the devil an inch.*** Overshadow him by praising God—even when you are hurting. One thing that the enemy can't stand is for you to find joy in the middle of your problems. That's why the Bible says, *"Delight yourself in the Lord, and you shall have the desires of your heart"* (Psalm 37:4). Rejoice in God and give thanks. Add praise to your treatment plan.

5. ***Faith is more than a mental attitude.*** It is action. Do things that encourage your faith. Find ways to express faith in the God who heals us. Sometimes something as simple as walking a few steps is an act of faith. Pursuing your normal routine in the face of pain is an act of faith. Put your faith into action.

6. ***Words and health are connected.*** Thinking and speaking positively about your situation promotes healing. The Bible says that life and death are in the tongue (Prov. 18:21). As a person thinks in his heart, so is he (Prov. 23:7). Jesus spoke the word and healed people. Positive thoughts and words will enhance

your medical treatment—and work to bring your healing.

7. *Don't allow symptoms to determine your state of health.* The job of a doctor is to find symptoms and trace them back to a cause. There's nothing wrong with that. But don't stay focused on your symptoms. They will always point toward sickness. Focus instead on signs that show you are getting better. Dwelling on negative thoughts will keep you sick. Before Israel decided to enter the Promised Land, they sent a few men to spy out the land (Num. 13:31-33). Though the land flowed with milk and honey, it was filled with giants and warriors, too. The Bible says that the people of Israel thought of themselves as grasshoppers before the giants who held the land. And they never ate the milk and honey. As long as we think that way about our health, we won't get well. In fact, we won't even fight if we believe that our disease is greater than the resources we have to overcome it.

8. *Do not spend time comparing your illness with the illness of someone who has died.* Don't ask how someone else got sick. Don't focus on losing the battle against disease. The Apostle Paul said, "If there be anything good, think on it" (Phil 4:8). Share the goodness of God with your family and friends. Talk about good health and the things that God has done for you. Meditate on the promises of God for your healing. Fill your mind with positive things. Your life is at stake.

9. *Develop good relationships.* Positive relationships and the comfort of loved ones bring us health. Find a community of love and prayer. A part of the community of faith is leadership that you can trust. The Bible says, "Is anyone among you sick? Let him call for the elders of the church, and let them pray over him, anointing him with oil in the name of the Lord. And the prayer of faith will save the sick, and the *Lord will raise him up*" (James 5:14-15). Our involvement in community is vital to helping us get well.

THREE

The Wholeness That Comes Through Jesus Christ

The Wholeness of God

Few words are as evocative of well-being as "wholeness." But what does wholeness really mean? And how can we actually achieve it? The answers to these questions make a difference in the quality of our lives. But even more importantly, they make a difference in how we view God and what we receive from Him.

Wholeness is a healthy, happy, and emotionally balanced life where there is no lack. God wants us to live in health and to prosper. Yet many of us fall sick and suffer. Why? There are no easy answers to the question of human suffering. Anyone who would tell you otherwise has either never reflected profoundly on the human condition or never experienced real suffering personally. The question becomes even more complex when we address it with the faith that God is loving and compassionate and seeks our good.

These are not new questions. The Bible addresses those who believe that God is delaying judgment and thereby allowing evil to prosper. The writer states emphatically that what seems like "slackness" to some is, in fact, God's longsuffering, which brings salvation to us (2 Peter 3:9). God does not want anyone to perish apart from Him; instead He desires that everyone should repent and find salvation. The writer is not implying that all *will* be saved, but that God's *desire* is for everyone to be saved. The point is that God's will interacts with our freedom. We must choose God's gracious offer of salvation despite circumstances that sometimes make us think that evil has the advantage over good.

This same interaction of God's will and our freedom helps us to frame our understanding of sickness and suffering. God also desires that everyone be in good health and prosper, though clearly we do not always experience God's wholeness. Many of us are sick, and suffering is a part of human existence. It comes down to the misuse of our freedom, whether we sin as an individual or as a society. This sin creates a negative cumulative effect on our environment and the world in which we live—which allows sickness and suffering to flourish despite God's will for our wholeness.

God did not want it to be that way. God created humanity to live in wholeness. But God also created us to live in freedom. It is as timeless as the story of what happened in the Garden of Eden. When we used our freedom to listen to the voice of Satan instead of the command of God, humanity was subjected to pain and suffering and death (Gen. 3:10-19). But God's will for wholeness still stands—in the midst of Satan's rebellion and our disobedience. In some ways, the gospel message is as simple as the old signs that used to appear on churches all over the South: "Jesus Saves." Through Jesus, God is restoring us to the wholeness for which He created us in the first place. Jesus is the door to experiencing God's wholeness—not just in heaven, not just in some glorious future day, but even now, in spite of the sickness and suffering that beset us.

God's Times and Methods

God heals us in many ways. When injured or diseased, our bodies actually work to heal themselves naturally—without any other kind of intervention. Regular exercise and good nutrition simply help the body to do its job. When needed, doctors and other medical professionals should be seen as partners who get involved in the healing process. Both the body's natural efforts to heal itself and the benefits we receive from medical science are gifts from God. Beyond these healing gifts, however, God also heals us through miracles. Miraculous healing is an undeniable sign that God has stepped into our lives supernaturally, demonstrating His power over the forces of sin and disease that trouble us.[1]

No doubt there are some reading this book who are suffering from many other kinds of illness besides cancer. Many are waiting for medical science to find new treatments and cures. Others are hoping some new herb will be found to alleviate their problems. Still others are looking for a miracle. We are all seeking something to move us from sickness to health, from illness to well-being. And all of us have obstacles that must be overcome in order for us to find the healing we seek, whether it's a lack of money or support or faith. But there is a moment—a place and time—when we must make the move for ourselves. We have to do something to move into that place of well-being for which we long.

The Gospel of John tells an insightful story about a man who had been sick for a very long time (5:1-14). The man stayed near a pool of water, along with many others who were sick, waiting for an angel to come who "troubled the waters." They believed that the first to get into the water after the angel touched it would be cured. But this opportunity for healing had become an excuse for the man: someone else always got there first. Jesus asked the man a simple, challenging question: "Do you want to be made well?" Then he commanded the sick man to get up, take his mat, and walk. The man was healed.

We often miss God's opportunities for healing. It is far easier than we may want to admit for us to become used to being sick. Whether the waters are troubled or Jesus walks up to your sickbed, you must recognize when God is present to heal. When we are "on the look out" for God's presence, anticipating opportunities for healing, we move from an attitude of resignation to a spirit of expectation. Many times, in fact, our expectation that God is about to act helps create an atmosphere of faith, opening the door for the Spirit of God to move in our lives.

Recognizing when God is present to heal is very different from trying to force God in a box that says there is only one way He can heal us. We must know that God wants to make us whole and expect Him to do it. But that is not at all the same thing as demanding that God operate according to some preconceived idea of how and when healing should take place. The only pattern that we can follow with confidence is what we see in the Word of God. If we take time to examine the many ways Jesus healed, we will realize that He exercised a lot of freedom in the methods He used to heal. Sometimes He touched the sick with His hands and then prayed. Other times, He just spoke a word. On occasion, He healed by casting out demons. One time He spat on clay and put it in the eyes of a blind man. He told a group of lepers to show themselves to the priests. And once He even prayed for a man twice. My point is not that you need to look for the strange and unusual in order to find God's power to heal. What I am saying is that God's power to make you whole can't be found in prepackaged formulas. When we lock God in a box, we could very well miss where He is present to heal us—perhaps in a surprising way.

If we are going to take advantage of God's opportunities for wholeness, we must decide to live according to what we believe, not by what we see or feel. I know that's easier said than done. I've been down the same road that you, or perhaps a friend or a family member, is traveling right now. I know how hard it is to think of having a good day when you've been hurting for so long, when what you used to consider a "normal" day is just a blurry memory. I understand it because I've lived it. But let me encourage you. No day is ever bad when we focus on the promise of Jesus to give us abundant life (John 10:10). Jesus Christ is hope. If we don't choose to live with that faith and hope, all that we have left is despair.

Jesus did not die on the cross just to save your soul from hell. He gave His life to open the way for a new dimension of living for us on earth, as well as a new dimension of living for us in heaven. Our salvation means that Jesus has taken us into His victory. Healing is an important part of that salvation. God is the author of healing for the total person. Salvation means our spirits are reborn, our minds renewed, and our bodies healed. I firmly believe that now is the time to realize that we do not have to live in a dimension of heartache and sorrow, but we can live in a realm of victory.

Steps for the Pursuit of Wholeness

1. *Have faith.* Faith is the trust we put in a God who can do anything—even create a universe out of nothing. Faith is the conviction that God will triumph over evil. Why? Because we know that Jesus Christ has already overcome the forces of darkness by His death on the cross and the power of His resurrection from the dead. This faith saves you, and this faith will heal you. Trusting God empowers us to dare—and to achieve—what might oth-

erwise seem impossible for us. The opposite of faith is a doubting uncertainty that crumbles in despair and hopelessness before adversity. Genuine faith, however, is not afraid of any circumstance. Faith never gives up. When uncertainty is replaced by this kind of faith, what once was impossible becomes possible. Until we believe that there is a Promised Land, we will never inherit it. Until we believe that God wants to give us wholeness, we will never receive it. Develop your faith in God, one step at a time—learning daily to trust His character and goodness. James exhorts us, *"But let him ask in faith, with no doubting, for he who doubts is like a wave of the sea driven and tossed by the wind. For let not that man suppose that he will receive anything from the Lord; he is a double-minded man, unstable in all his ways"* (1:6-8).

2. *Encourage yourself.* The Bible says that David "strengthened himself" in the Lord (I Samuel 30:6). He found the strength to praise God, even in the most devastating moments of his life. Yet through his example, we learn an important truth: it is precisely when it is

hardest to see God that we most need to seek Him. We cannot allow depression over our illness to darken our whole world. We must choose to praise God despite our troubles. Have a discipline of prayer and meditation. Take God's Word and memorize it, especially scriptures that will uplift you: *"All things are possible to him who believes"* (Mark 9:23) or *"Delight yourself also in the Lord, and He shall give you the desires of your heart"* (Psalm 37:4). Surround yourself with family and friends, people that love you and give life to you. Press yourself to maintain normal activities and responsibilities. Maintain social commitments. Exercise appropriately, and stick to a healthy diet. These are all ways that we can follow David's example and encourage ourselves. When we do, we will cultivate a positive attitude about what God is doing in our lives.

3. *Educate yourself about your condition.* Get information on available resources that might help you. Never be afraid to ask questions. Through ignorance we become our own worst enemy. Take the time to research; find

out what the medical community is saying, as well as the experience of others fighting the same disease. If we are well-informed, we will be able to make an educated decision regarding the best treatment for our condition. Find out about experimental and alternative approaches, as well as conventional treatments. Don't settle for any treatment until you are convinced that you know absolutely everything you need to know about it. Get a second and third opinion, if necessary. (At the end of this book, I have included a section outlining resources that will be of help to you.)

4. *Believe in God's report.* At every turn, you will be bombarded with information about your disease. You may even be overwhelmed by the facts concerning your particular diagnosis. But it is God's truth—not medical facts—that sets you free. Truth is a lot more than just the sum total of all the facts you can amass about a given circumstance. Truth is how God sees the matter. That doesn't mean you have to be in a state of denial. Denial is nothing more than fear of the

facts. Knowing the truth simply means the facts don't have the last word. We must soberly recognize our problem, to be sure. At the same time, however, we must not allow a bad report—based on the facts—to control our future. When I found out I was sick, my concern at that point was fighting cancer, but the truth spoken through the prophetic word by Pastor Tommy Reid gave me hope. Having faith in Jesus means that you are convinced beyond the testimony of your present circumstance that victory is in Christ. Not one scripture says evil will overcome good. Good wins—always. Meditate on God's promises found in the Bible; these promises are God's Word to you personally. The Word of God is living and powerful, sharper than a double-edged sword (Heb. 4:12). That living, powerful sword is your weapon against the forces of depression and defeat. Say in your heart, "God, if you'll do your part, I'll do mine." Then watch God work.

5. *Make good decisions.* God takes decision-making very seriously. When Jesus went to the Garden of Gesthemane before His be-

trayal, He was prayerfully making a decison about the will of God for His life (Luke 22:42). When there is a decision that will determine the rest of your life, don't take it lightly. Pride, self-deception, and ignorance are just a few of the obstacles to making a good decision. Before making any decision, however, be sure to get all the facts first. Once you have the facts, take them before God and seek spiritual counseling. Find out what God says about the matter. Search for biblical principles that can help guide you in the specific choices you must make. Don't feel pressured to make a quick decision. Always keep in mind that once we make a decision, we are the ones responsible for it. When all is said and done, the life you have is your own. Others are there only to help and encourage you—even your physicians. Be studious about your decisions—diligently evaluating competent counsel. Seek God, and then trust that you have the wisdom you need to discern the best options for your situation.

6. *Realize that destiny is a gift God has placed within every human being.* We don't really

know who we are until we discover God's destiny for our lives. God wants you to understand His plan for your life and to succeed in your life's mission. You are created by God and chosen by Him to fulfill a very specific destiny. What you consider to be limitations cannot restrict you, if you give yourself completely to God's destiny for your life. God told Abraham that he would have a child in his old age. Because he had more regard for God's promise than his physical limitations, the Bible says that Abraham "did not consider his own body." Check the direction that you are going. Ask the Lord to order your steps every day. And be focused. The Bible tells us Jesus "set his face" to go to Jerusalem (Luke 9:51). No one was going to turn Him aside from His destiny. It tells us that Paul was determined to go where He knew his destiny beckoned him. He said, "I must go to Rome" (Acts 19:21). Set your face toward the wholeness that God intends for you.

7. *Have a reason to be well.* It is vital that we feel we have a reason to live. If you want to

be whole, discover your destiny—and your purpose. I believe there is a subtle but meaningful difference between destiny and purpose. Destiny is the ultimate intention for which God created us. Purpose, however, has to do with the goals that we set for ourselves. Each goal points toward our ultimate destiny. For example, Joseph's destiny was to save Israel during famine, but his purpose was to be obedient and humble in the various circumstances he encountered along the way. Once we discover the destiny for which God created us, we must find purpose in life. Don't lose sight of your goals—whether they are long-term or short-term. Cultivate and nourish the desire to be well in order to fulfill your destiny and to accomplish your purpose. There will be mountains you will cast into the sea by faith and others you will climb by faith. There will be times you may wonder if you can make it through one more day. But even then, in your darkest moments, keep pressing. Your goal is just within reach.

---

[1]Earl Paulk and Dan Rhodes, *A Theology for the Next Millennium* (Georgia, Earl Paulk Ministries, 2000)

FOUR

Spiritual Laws of Healing

The Spiritual Laws of Healing

I'll be the first to admit that there are many things about God we just don't know. That's because He's infinite. And we're finite. He has no beginning and end. We have both: we're born, and one day we'll die. There is so much more to God than we can possibly comprehend with our limited minds. God is simply "bigger" than our small thoughts can hold. But, fortunately, that's not the end of the story. God desires a relationship with us. Since it's hard to relate to a mystery, God graciously reveals Himself to us. His revelation comes in many ways: through the world around us, through other people, through our own conscience. And, of course, one of our primary sources of knowledge about God is through the pages of Scripture. But God's most important revelation to us is Jesus. When we see Jesus, we see God. We see His character and will completely expressed in the life of one human being. By taking God's revelation of Himself to us, we can discern patterns and develop principles—laws—that show how God relates to us. And God has revealed several laws that affect our health.

The Law of Faith

It may sound strange, but God is not *obligated* to heal us outside of a personal relationship of faith. And it's not just our faith that God recognizes. God sometimes heals us because of the faith He sees in our friends or loved ones. In fact, faith is such a powerful factor in healing that even Jesus could do only a few miracles in His own hometown because of their lack of faith (Luke 4:23-27). Does that mean that God *cannot* heal us without faith? Of course not. Remember, we're not trying to lock God into a box: "God only heals if..." We are just trying to discern God's patterns of healing. The simple fact is that God chooses to use our faith as a channel through which He brings healing into our lives. Faith is a lot more than just a positive mental attitude. It's more than a set of dogmatic beliefs to which we're committed. Faith is personal. Faith is trust. Faith is our part of a relationship with God.

The Law of Covenant

Another principle of healing is the law of covenant. Covenant is a strange word to modern ears. It's not a word that we use very much any more. But it's a very important word in the Bible. And like faith, it has to do with our relationship with God. The closest example that we might understand today is the covenant of marriage. In marriage, two people enter into a special relationship with one another by making vows and promises to each other. They maintain that special relationship by living out those vows and keeping those promises. That's covenant. Covenant gives us insight into the way that God sees His relationship with us. In fact, the very first promise God gave concerning healing and protection from disease flowed out of a covenant relationship between God and His people in the Old Testament (Exodus 15:26).. We keep our covenant with God by obeying His commands from our heart. There's no question whether God will keep His part of the covenant. He's faithful, even when we're unfaithful. We must come to understand, however, that our faithfulness to covenant is one of the principles that clears the way for us to receive healing.

The Law of Structure

Another way God heals is through the law of structure. Make no mistake about it, God doesn't create chaos or bring confusion. He fixes it. God wants to bring order and peace. God has set a structure—a care system—through which He provides healing. That's what Jesus did when He gave His disciples the authority to heal. Jesus delegated His authority to heal through a visible structure that could reach others. Whether it's a parent praying for a sick child or a pastor caring for a parishioner, God works through structure. James instructs us to call for the elders of the church when we are sick so that they can pray for us to be healed (5:14). And God responds. Why? God entrusts His authority to human beings. When we recognize and respect the authority that God puts within a structure, we demonstrate our implicit respect for God's own authority. We prove that we are not the ultimate authority in our lives—that we are not our own god. Just like the Roman centurion who came to Jesus and asked only that Jesus say the word, those who understand authority recognize the authority that God exercises over all things—including sickness (Matt. 8:8).

The Law of God's Higher Purposes

If we're going to make sense out of God's thoughts about healing at all, then we must come back to the point where we started. God is bigger than our thoughts. No matter what we might think is best, God is the One who ultimately knows best. Sometimes that's a hard truth for us to accept. But it demands that we trust God. The bottom line is that God is the One who heals, not us. God knows more than we do. And God loves us more than we could ever love even our dearest loved one—or our own selves. God reserves the right to heal those whom He wills according to His higher purposes and what is ultimately best for the individual. So what are we supposed to do? Are we just to fold our hands and hope everything works out all right? If you think that, then you've missed the whole point of this book. God calls us to earnestly pray for those who need healing (Job 42:7-10). He asks that we speak words of encouragement and hope to those who despair of life. We know that we have to take up the fight against the works of the devil. And that's a fight we'll always win. In God's game plan, death isn't defeat. Nor should it bring fear. For those who trust God, life doesn't end when our bodies die. Life always triumphs over death.

Miracles Take Place at the End of Human Possibilities

So what about miracles? The truth is we don't think a lot about miracles until we need one. Miracles show the power of God over sickness and evil. They also show that God is willing to get involved in our lives when we have nothing else we can do. Miracles don't happen until there is a crisis that requires God to step in. The Bible tells a story about a woman who needed a miracle (Mark 5:22-26). The woman had suffered from a flow of blood for twelve years. She had done everything she knew to do. She had gone to the doctors. She had spent all her money. And she only got worse. Certainly this woman was a candidate for a miracle. So why doesn't every desperate person get a miracle? A hopeless situation may set us up for a miracle, but it takes more than that. The woman believed God could do something for her if she did her part. She said in her heart, "If only I could touch Jesus' garment, I'll be made well." And that's exactly what she did. She had to fight her way through the crowd before she could get close to Jesus. But she did it. And as a result, what doctors couldn't do and money wouldn't buy, God healed by a miracle. No, I can't give you five easy steps to a guaranteed miracle. But I can give you guidelines that will help in your pursuit of healing.

Creating the Atmosphere for Miracles

The woman who touched Jesus' garment helped to create an atmosphere for a miracle by her faith. We have the same responsibility. So how do we set the stage for God to do the impossible in our lives? We have to get in the Spirit. John said in the Book of Revelation that he was "in the Spirit on the Lord's day" (Rev. 1:10). We can't be ruled by the flesh and ruled by the Spirit at the same time. Being open to the Spirit of God means being receptive to God's will for your life. It means knowing God wants to make you whole. It means encouraging your faith in what God can do in you. Both fasting and prayer can help us move beyond the flesh and become open to the Spirit in our lives. When we are ruled by the flesh, however, we are controlled by our reason, our instinct, and by our own understanding. We refuse to give God the freedom to work with us in His way. We lock God into the box we've made for Him.

But creating an atmosphere for miracles means learning to press beyond your limits—whether they are self-imposed or forced on us by sickness. We can live in the Spirit with such confidence that the impossible becomes possible. It's in this dimension of living above our limits that we experience God's power. Jesus demonstrated it. And He has given us the same power through the gift of the Holy Spirit.

Igniting Your Miracle

While God is the source of miracles, we have to do our part. Many times when Jesus healed, the faith of those to whom He ministered ignited the release of the Spirit's power. Faith gives God glory even before our eyes see it. There are many ways to release God's power. It is important to seek God's presence. Yes, God is everywhere, but we must start looking for the places where He is moving. We release God's power by challenging the pain or the fear that seeks to destroy us. Don't compromise with disease. Demand nothing less than unconditional surrender. Use your mouth to declare God's Word over your life. Others will tell you how well the disease is doing. Tell yourself how well God is doing. If we are going to release God's power, we need to take what we have, whatever that might be, and give it back to God so that He can turn it into a miracle. Let God show Himself strong in your weaknesses.

My own personal experience has led me to the conclusion that when we give our lives to God, He will give us the strength we need to finish our course. As long as God has a job left for us to do, He will keep us healthy enough to finish it. That means we should seek God and His will for our lives, rather than just seeking healing for its own sake. When we are unsure of God's will for us, we need to do what Jesus did in the Garden of Gethsemane (Matt. 26:39-42). After praying that the cup of death would pass from Him, He realized that God had summoned Him to a destiny higher than His own will. We can find the same peace He possessed, and the same strength of God to carry us toward our destiny, when we pray as He did, "Not my will, God, but Your will be done."

FIVE

Oh! It's Just You, Cancer

Cancer: The Most Feared Word

This generation is more oriented to staying in good health than any other generation before it. We live in a day of tremendous medical resources and knowledge. Yet, every year more than one million Americans hear their doctors say the words we have come to fear more than any others: "You have cancer." For many of us, this diagnosis seems like a virtual death sentence. This is true, in spite of the fact that half of the more than eight million Americans alive today with a history of cancer can consider themselves cured, while the other half is undergoing treatment to be cured.

A cancer diagnosis presents many challenges. For most of us, cancer is something that happens to someone else. We hear a lot about cancer, sure, but the reality is that we're never really prepared to face it. The sad fact is that with all of our increased awareness of cancer, our actual knowledge of what is taking place in our bodies or in the bodies of someone we love is almost nonexistent. When we are diagnosed with cancer, we are challenged emotionally, financially, physically, mentally, and spiritually—all at once. We face a seemingly unending list of confusing treatment options. In an instant, our attitude about cancer changes. No longer do we anxiously wonder, "Will it happen to me?" Now we begin to ask ourselves and our doctors, "What can I do about it?"

What Is Cancer?

Cancer is a combination of related diseases. It involves the malfunction of genes that control cell growth and division.

Normal body cells multiply, divide, and then die in an orderly fashion. From conception, normal cells begin dividing to produce growth. As the body develops and matures, this process slows down. Once it reaches adulthood, the normal cells of most tissues divide only to replace dying cells or to repair injuries.

Cancer cells, however, continue to radically grow and divide and even spread to other parts of the body. As they accumulate, they form *tumors* (lumps) that may compress, invade, and destroy surrounding tissue. If these abnormal cells break away from such a tumor, they can travel through the bloodstream or the lymph system to other areas of the body. Once there, they may settle and form "colony" tumors—which, in turn, continue to grow and spread. This spread of a tumor to a new site is called *metastasis.*

Cancer is classified by its appearance under a microscope and by the part of the body from which it originated. Each type of cancer varies in how it grows and spreads. Generally, the more abnormal (in medical terms, *undifferentiated*) the cells look under the microscope, the more malignant or serious the cancer is. When cells are greatly undifferentiated, the cancer is likely to be more active and less controllable. No matter where it spreads, the cancer is still labeled after the part where it began.

For example, if prostate cancer spreads to the bones, it is still prostate cancer, or if colon cancer spreads to the kidney, it is still labeled colon cancer.

Cancer is caused by both internal factors (hormones, immune conditions, and inherited mutations) and external factors (chemicals, radiation, and viruses). By acting together or in sequence, these factors may initiate or promote the inception of cancer. Often ten or more years will pass between the exposures or mutations and any detectable cancer.

It is important to realize that not all tumors are cancerous. Benign (noncancerous) tumors usually can be permanently removed and do not spread to other parts of the body. Most of the time, they are not considered life threatening unless they are growing in a confined area, such as the brain.[1]

What Is Cancer Staging?

Once a cancer is found, multiple tests will be preformed to determine its stage. Based on the primary tumor's size and location in the body, as well as any spreading that may have occurred, this will help to describe the extent of the disease within the body. Different staging systems are used to classify cancerous tumors. The *TNM staging system* stands for: (T) the condition of the primary tumor including the level of invasion, (N) any lymph node involvement, and (M) any sign of metastasis. Once these are accessed, a *stage* of I, II, III or IV is assigned—Stage I being barely detectable to Stage IV being extremely aggressive and spreading. *Summary staging* may also be used in describing the tumor. An "in situ" stage is used if the cancer is only in the layer of cells where it originally developed without any spreading. If the cancer cells have spread beyond that original layer, then the cancer is labeled "invasive"—whether local, regional, or distant.

Who Can Get Cancer?

Anyone is susceptible—regardless of age, race or gender. According to the American Cancer Society, half of all men and one-third of all women in the United States will develop cancer over the course of a lifetime. Today, there are literally millions of people around the world who are either living with cancer or have already been cured of the disease.

What is a Risk Factor?

A *risk factor* is anything that increases the chance of developing a disease such as cancer. Risk factors can vary among different types of cancer, but they can also share similarities. For example, smoking increases the risk of cancer for many areas, including the lungs, mouth, throat, larynx, and bladder; while leaving the skin unprotected in strong sunlight increases the risk for skin cancer. These factors do put a person at greater risk, but they do not always "cause" the disease. Many people with one or more risk factors never develop cancer; others who develop cancer have no known risk factors. However, it is still important to be aware of the factors involved and then to take appropriate action—whether that means changing your behavior or being monitored closely for a potential cancer.

Cancer Treatments

The array of treatments and therapies now available to those dealing with a cancerous condition can be confusing and overwhelming. Some treatments seem remarkably successful; others are still in the exploratory stages, while still others can be even more damaging to the body. Each option comes with its own set of conditions—both good and bad. Unfortunately, nothing is entirely risk-free.

The following is a brief explanation of the terms used to classify general cancer treatments:[2]

Proven: This is a mainstream medical treatment that has undergone thorough testing under a strict set of guidelines. Based on the evidence found, it has been proven to be safe and effective. The results are published in various journals which are reviewed by other doctors or scientists in the field. For example, radiation has already been widely used for many years. The Food and Drug Administration has approved this type of treatment.

Research or Investigational: These treatments are still being studied under clinical trial. They are considered experimental methods because they have not been fully tested. The first phase of research involves laboratory and animal testing. If the therapy is found safe and promising, actual patients become involved in the process—as with certain types of chemotherapy. Only when it is proven safe and effective on these patients will the Food and Drug Administration consider approving it for regular use. It is then that the treatment can become part of the standard, mainstream collection of proven therapies for treating a given disease.

Complementary: These supportive methods are recommended for use alongside mainstream treatments—not as substitutes. While they are not considered a part of curing the disease, they do help control symptoms and improve overall well being. Examples include meditation, massage therapy, and herbs.

Integrative Therapy: This term refers to the use of both mainstream and complementary therapies together in the treatment of a given disease.

Unproven or Untested: These terms are sometimes unclear in definition. Often they are used in reference to treatments with minimal scientific basis. They may also refer to those currently under investigation. Whatever the case, adequate evidence is not yet available. As always, it is important to use common sense and to do your own research.

Alternative: These treatments are normally promoted as cancer "cures." Yet, most have never been scientifically tested, or they have been tested but found to be ineffective. Some treatments that have been tested and found useless, such as laetrile, are renamed and repackaged and put back on the shelf. When these alternatives are *substituted* for proven treatments, additional pain and suffering may be incurred due to lack of adequate treatment or other harmful consequences.

Quackery: This term refers to the promotion of methods that dishonestly claim to prevent, diagnose, and even cure cancer or other serious diseases. Some promoters even engage in unethical sales techniques, charge unreasonable fees, make misleading promises and neglect prudent conventional medical supervision and care. Since there is usually little scientific evidence, select patient testimonials are primarily used in support of these unfounded methods.

Considerations for Cancer Treatments

1. **Consider the claims made for the treatment.**
   • Does it enable mainstream methods to work more successfully?
   • Will it relieve symptoms or side effects?
   • Is it based on an unproven theory?

- Does it claim to completely cure cancer and discourage you from using any conventional medical treatment?
- If used instead of standard therapies and clinical trials, will the resulting delay affect the chances for cure or advance the cancer stage?

2. **Consider the credentials of its supporters.**
   - Are they recognized experts in cancer treatment?
   - Have they published their findings in trustworthy journals?
   - Do they attack the medical/scientific establishment?
   - Is it primarily promoted through mass media—books, periodicals, TV and radio?

3. **Consider the total cost involved.**
   - Does it require you to travel out of the country.

4. **Consider the availability and usage.**
   - Is it accessible for wide-spread use within the health-care community?
   - Is it considered a "secret" with only limited availability?

It is important to carefully consider all of your choices—both through extensive research and personal references. Each type of cancer reacts differently to various kinds of treatments. Make sure you find medical professionals you can trust and keep them as a part of your decision-making process. Together you can carefully combine a variety of treatments that will bring the best results in your situation.

The Reality of Prevention

Cancer is not necessarily inevitable. In fact, it is often preventable. Inherited genetics is a factor, but the development of cancer is largely due to other more controllable issues. Although not enough is known to prevent all cancers entirely, we now know more than ever before about the reality of prevention. You can take control of your health and play an active role in reducing your risk.

Scientific evidence suggests that approximately one-third of cancer-related deaths in the United States each year are due to tobacco usage, with another third due to dietary factors. Basically that means most of these deaths could be *entirely* prevented by simple lifestyle changes. Of course, nothing can guarantee full protection against any disease. Yet, the introduction of healthful practices at any stage from childhood to old age can promote health and reduce cancer risk.

Based on the findings of the American Cancer Society and the American Institute for Cancer Research, certain guidelines have been established. These are consistent with the US Department of Agriculture (USDA) Food Guide Pyramid (1992), the Dietary Guidelines for Americans (1995) and the dietary recommendations of various other agencies. They have been compiled based on the analysis of more than 4,500 research studies done by the American Institute for Cancer Research. Basically, there are three areas of concern: dietary practices, physical activity, and healthy habits.[3]

GUIDELINES FOR DIETARY PRACTICES

1. *Most of the foods you eat should come from plant sources.* It is important to choose a wide variety of vegetables and fruits—at least

five servings each day. Many scientific studies show that eating fruits and vegetables (especially green and dark yellow vegetables and those in the cabbage family, soy products, and legumes) gives added protection against cancers —especially in the gastrointestinal and respiratory tracts. It is also good to include other foods from plant sources such as breads, cereals, grain products, rice, pasta, and beans. Grains provide many vitamins and minerals such as foliate, calcium, and selenium, which have been associated with lowering the risk of colon cancer.

2. *Limit your portions of food from animal sources.* Meats should be eaten in moderation. Consumption of meats, especially red meat, has been associated with increased cancer risk particularly in the colon and prostate. When eaten, red meat should be limited to 80 grams (3 ounces) daily. Fish, poultry, and meat from non-domesticated animals should be chosen more often.

3. *Watch all the extras.* The key is in prepara-
tion. Foods eaten in their most natural state
are going to yield healthier benefits. This
means to avoid overcooked food. This also
means to choose fresh or frozen vegetables
and fruits over those canned. Less process-
ing means more nutritional value. It is especially important to limit fat, refined sugar,
and salt—which can sometimes be hidden
in processed foods. When preparing meals,
use herbs and spices to season foods. Also,
choose modest amounts of appropriate veg-
etable oils—primarily extra virgin olive oil.
High-fat diets have been associated with a
heightened risk of cancers of the colon, rectum, prostate and endometrium. Also note
that when properly regulated, additives, con-
taminants, and other residues in food and
drink are not known to be harmful. However, unregulated or improper use can be a
health hazard—especially in developing
countries.

4. *Ensure proper preservation of foods.* Only
eat foods that have been stored properly.
Perishable foods should be refrigerated and

maintained at proper temperatures. It is not recommended to eat any food which is liable to contamination with mycotoxins due to prolonged storage at ambient temperatures.

GUIDELINES FOR PHYSICAL ACTIVITY

1. *Pursue physical activities each day.* Physical activity is important to maintain good health as well as to provide protection against disease. If your work schedule is primarily sedentary, it is especially important to engage in some type of physical exercise for at least an hour each day. This could be a brisk walk, a bicycle ride, or any similar activity.

2. *Incorporate vigorous physical activity at least once a week.* For all, vigorous exercise is recommended for at least one hour per week. The proper balance of caloric intake and energy expenditure is necessary to achieve and maintain a healthy body weight.

It is important not to be underweight or over-weight—limiting weight gain during adult-hood to less than 5 kg (11 pounds). Obesity can increase the risk for cancer , including those in the colon, rectum, prostate, en-dometrium, breast, and kidney.

GUIDELINES FOR HEALTHY HABITS

1. *Stay away from alcohol and tobacco.* It is highly recommended to refrain from drink-ing alcoholic beverages, as well as smoking or chewing tobacco. If consumed, alcoholic drinks should be limited to less than two drinks a day for men and one a day for women.

2. *Always protect yourself from the sun.* It is expected that over one million cases of skin cancer will be diagnosed in the next year. Many could have been easily prevented with adequate protection from the sun's rays.

3. *Ensure regular examinations.* For cancers of the breast and skin, self-examinations can result in detection of tumors at an early stage. However, the best way to ensure detection of any cancerous situation is to schedule regular check-ups with a health care professional. Usually the most effective strategy is a combination of two or more early detection approaches (such as breast self-examination, mammography, and clinical breast examination by a doctor). The sooner a cancer is found, the sooner treatments can begin—which can not only save lives but also reduce suffering. A cancer-related checkup is recommended every three years for those from the ages of twenty to forty and then annually for those forty and older. Depending on a person's age, this might include examinations for cancers of the thyroid, oral cavity, skin, lymph nodes, testes, and ovaries, as well as for various nonmalignant diseases. This appointment should include health counseling as well as a thorough examination.

---

[1] The American Cancer Society Website (www.cancer.org)

[2] The American Cancer Society Website (www.cancer.org)

[3] The American Cancer Society Website (www.cancer.org)

SIX

Prostate Cancer

My Personal Experience

At least twenty years ago, I became aware that I had an enlarged prostate. As you may know, this condition is common as men grow older. My doctor monitored the condition of my prostate in yearly physical exams. It was not until the late 1980's, however, as my PSA count started to rise, that the doctor recommended a biopsy. I continued to have biopsies on my prostate performed fairly regularly until 1998. But when my PSA count jumped to 230, I was admitted to the hospital for a series of more in-depth biopsies. It was then that I was diagnosed with cancer. If cancer had been discovered earlier, treatment would have been much more simple, but now drastic action had to be taken. Several glands around my prostate were removed, and I began to take Lupron, a hormonal treatment. In addition to all this, I underwent two months of radiation treatment at a local clinic.

Why am I telling you this? Because I want to urge all men to have regular check-ups as they pass the age of forty. If cancer can be diagnosed early enough, there are more and better methods of dealing with it, such as implanting radiation seeds in the prostate or, in some cases, removing the prostate itself.

Treatment has brought my PSA count down considerably. However, through the prayers of many around the world, including Benny Hinn, my PSA count has been reduced to 1.1 at the writing of this book. Undoubtedly, this is not only acceptable, but excellent. Of course, I will continue to monitor my progress, as I have done in the past. But in all things, I give God the glory.

Prostate Cancer Testing

In the beginning stages of prostate cancer, there are usually no symptoms evident. As with any cancerous situation, a combination of methods can ensure prostate tumors are detected at the onset when they are most likely to be cured. The two most common are the *PSA test* and the *digital rectal examination.* The PSA test is a blood test for prostate-specific antigen—which is a protein produced by the prostate gland. When heightened, it can signal that an abnormal condition is present. The digital rectal examination can also be done as a part of any routine physical examination. This method allows the doctor to feel the prostate gland for irregularities. It is extremely important for men over the age of forty to have these particular examinations done each year. For those who are at a higher risk, testing should begin even earlier.[1]

Depending on these findings, further testing may be needed to make a definitive diagnosis. These will usually begin with an ultrasound screening and biopsy where pieces of tissue are taken from the prostate and examined under the microscope. Again, depending on the outcome, other techniques may be utilized. These may include a prostatic acid phosphatase (PAP) test, urinalysis, cystoscopy, bone scan, computerized tomography (CT) scan, lymph node analysis or magnetic resonance imaging (MRI).

PSA LEVELS and THEIR MEANING

LEVEL	MEANING
0-4 ng/ml	Normal level, depending on age -+
2.4 ng/ml	Normal for ages 41-50
3.5 ng/ml	Normal for ages 51-60
4.5 ng/ml	Normal for ages 61-70
6.5 ng/ml	Normal for ages 61-70
4-10 ng/ml	Moderated elevated
Over 10 ng/ml	High

Prostate Cancer Diagnosis

With the combined results of these tests, the status of the prostate and any cancer present can be seen. Most cases of prostate cancer, unlike many other cancers, do not progress rapidly. This allows for time to carefully weigh the options and make quality decisions. You need to fully understand your cancer diagnosis. Besides the PSA level, you will need to know the tumor size and volume, the location, the Gleason grade, the stage, and the pattern of growth.

The Gleason Grade

The Gleason grade is a method used to determine the variations of cells when a piece of tissue is examined under a microscope. The grade measures differentiation and indicates how closely cancer cells resemble their normal counterparts. Five different patterns of cells are recognized in this system and classified from 1 to 5—from closely packed and well within the tumor margin to wide-spread and infiltrating. One number is assigned to the most prominent pattern of the cells and another to the secondary pattern. The two totaled together make up the Gleason grade—which can range anywhere from 2 (1+1) to 10 (5+5).

GLEASON GRADES and THEIR MEANING

GRADE	MEANING
Gleason 2, 3, 4	Most like normal cells, well differentiated, slow growing, low probability of metastasis, low grade.
Gleason 5, 6, 7	Can behave like normal cells or like aggressive cells, moderately differentiated, moderate probability of metastasis, moderate grade.
Gleason 8, 9, 10	Least like normal cells, poorly differentiated, high probability of metastasis.

The Staging of Prostate Cancer

As previously discussed, there are several classifications used to stage cancer. The most common with prostate cancer is the TNM method using Stages I to IV. Stage I means the cancer is completely confined to the prostate and is still barely detectable—found only through a PSA test, ultrasound, or accidentally during surgery. When the tumor can be felt but is still confined to the prostate gland, it is labeled Stage II. Stage III indicates that the cancer has spread to tissues immediately surrounding the prostate. Finally, at Stage IV the cancer cells have been found in the lymph nodes or other organs and tissues outside the prostate.

All available factors should be considered when exploring cancer treatments. Of course, the larger and more aggressive the tumor, the quicker decisions must be made. A cancer is considered more threatening if the location of its original tumor is in the outer area (peripheral) rather than the inner (transitional) area. Symptoms, age, and other illnesses should also play a major role in making a good decision.

Prostate Cancer Treatments

As with any cancer, it is important that you and your loved ones know exactly what your options are. Your doctor should be someone you can trust to help you through this process. But don't stop there. Do your own research. So many new avenues are being explored in so many different places that you never know where you will find a clue to a treatment that may be helpful to you. If at all possible, get a second opinion before submitting to any type of treatment. There are doctors who specialize in treating cancer (oncologists). There are even specialists in every kind of cancer—down to the cell type. Seek out the opinion of someone who is dealing with your type of prostate cancer on a daily basis. It is also important to get a second pathological opinion. In the case of prostate cancer still in the early stages, it is usually difficult for doctors to know whether the cancer will progress and metastasize. This creates a dilemma and may lead to differences of opinion among health care professionals. In this instance, only you can ultimately determine which methods best suit you and your quality of life.

Some of the common proven methods that are used to treat prostate cancer include:

- **Prostatectomy:** An operation involving complete removal of the prostate.
- **External Radiation:** Radiation is delivered to the area in a linear acceleration. Usually, this radiation is given five times a week for a period of seven weeks.
- **Radiation Seeding:** Radioactive seeds are implanted in the prostate.

- **Hormonal Manipulation:** This deals with the male hormone testosterone. It is either eliminated by the removal of the testicles (or chiectomy) or suppressed by the injection of the Lupron hormone. It is commonly used prior to other treatment for removal of the prostate or when the cancer has advanced.

- **Watchful Waiting:** This kind of waiting may be used when the cancer is still considered Stage I. Older men who have decided that quality life is more important than the statistically short time that may be gained through aggressive therapy may also choose this option.

There are other treatments that are still considered in the investigative process:

- **Radiation Seeding (internal radiation or brachytherapy):** Radiation seeds are inserted into the prostate.

- **Cryosurgery:** The tissues of the prostate are destroyed by freezing techniques.

- **Chemotherapy:** A combination of drugs are given or implanted.

- **Hyperthermia:** Treating tumors by a variety of techniques employing heat, including microwaves.

Prostate Cancer: Questions and Answers

1. How common is prostate cancer?

Prostate cancer is the most commonly diagnosed cancer among men in the United States, excluding skin cancer. It is also the second leading cause of cancer death. The statistics report that one in five men have a lifetime risk of getting prostate cancer. That means a 40-year-old man's chance of getting prostate cancer in the next 10 years is one in 1,000. Over the next 20 years, it is one in 100 --- which is less than his risk of getting lung cancer.

2. Who can get it?

Any man is at risk for prostate cancer. There is still no way to completely ensure prevention. However, certain factors have been linked to an increased risk of developing this disease. Age is a major factor; more than 75 percent of all prostate cancers are diagnosed in men over age 65. The risk is greater for African-American men and for men with a history of the disease in their family. High-fat diets have also been linked to prostate cancer development. Studies are currently being done to see if a low-fat diet can reduce the risk.

3. Are there any symptoms?

Many times, men will not experience any type of symptoms at all before being diagnosed with prostate cancer. If they do, symptoms may include frequent urination or an inability to urinate, trouble starting or holding back the flow of urine, blood in the urine, and frequent pain or stiffness in the lower back, hips, pelvis or upper thighs. These symptoms may also signal a common, non-cancerous condition called Benign Prostatic Hyperplasia (BPH), which is simply an enlargement of the prostate gland. If any of these symptoms develop, it is important to seek immediate medical attention for proper diagnosis and treatment.

---

[1] Marion Morra & Eve Potts, *The Prostate Cancer Answer Book* (New York, Avon Books, 1996)

SEVEN

Wise As Serpents

Standing Against the Wiles of the Devil

Satan seeks to steal, kill, and destroy the life that Jesus has come to give us. He not only wants to steal your health—but he wants to take your peace of mind too. How we think is one of the most important keys to winning the battle against our adversary. As Jesus said, we must be wise as serpents but as innocent as doves. Today, many prominent leaders are under great physical attack. Oral Roberts, Robert Schuller, Billy Graham, Desmond Tutu, Andrew Young, Rudy Giuliani, and Bob Dole have all had recent health battles. With so many visible leaders under attack, we can wonder whether there is hope for us. But we must remember that God promises abundant life through Jesus Christ. Don't lose the battle for your body in your mind.

The Covenant of Your Mind

The following is an excerpt from another prophetic word Pastor Tommy Reid gave to me at the Cathedral. Because I believe it has great meaning for you as well, you can find it in its entirety at the end of this book.

"Here is a word God has specifically given me, and I have never seen this before, and I've never heard anyone say this before, but God so breathed into my spirit that I have to tell it to you. Your soul, your emotions, your mind, and your will shall know prosperity, because it says as your soul prospers. Let me tell you what I think this means: your mind shall know that covenant. Your mind is going to be filled with the greatest creative ideas that you have ever had—far beyond the creative ideas of your youth. Your mind shall know that covenant. Your mind will be filled with creative ideas that you have never heard before or seen before. Many times we look at those of us who are

older and wonder if we can be as creative as we were back in our past, but God is going to acti-vate the covenant of your mind—the prosperity of your mind."

I believe God wants to lift us to a dimension of living that Tommy Reid called the "covenant of the mind." But in order to do that, we must know the mind of Christ. There is a place in our relationship with God where we do not act out of our own emotion and will, but we do the will of the Father. We can live by the mind of Christ in our everyday lives. Just as Jesus did nothing of Himself, but made it clear that He acted out the will of His Heavenly Father, even so it should be the goal of every devoted Christian to follow the mind of Christ.

The Scriptures show that God is concerned about our minds. The Bible refers to various mindsets, or attitudes. Here are just a few:

- *The Anxious Mind* (Luke 12:29): God does not want us to be controlled by anxiety. Do not be fearful for what is taking place. The mind of Christ in us transcends our own worried emotions.

- *The Carnal Mind* (Colossians 2:18): This is a mind that cannot lift itself above the realm of the flesh into the realm of the Spirit. We must be led by the Spirit of God in order to overcome this attitude. The carnal mind sees the world only as it is measured by human standards.

- *The Double Mind* (James 1:8): A double mind is pulled in two conflicting directions, declaring complete loyalty to both. Like Peter, we declare we will die for Jesus, only later to deny we ever knew Him.

- *The Blinded Mind* (2 Corinthians 3:14): The "gods of this world," which Paul said are the ones responsible for blinding the minds of those who are lost, are gods whose base is pride. A blinded mind cannot see the world as God made it to be, only as we want it to be.

- *The Fair Mind* (Acts 17): We need to have a fair mind in our dealings with others. It reflects our attitude about others.

- *One Mind* (Romans 12:17): When we are in agreement, there is no way the enemy can defeat us. This is what the Bible means by one mind.

- *The Renewed Mind* (Romans 12:2): The human mind has been given over to sinful patterns of thinking since the fall of Adam. That is why it's important to renew our minds to God's original intention. Only then can we live out the will of God. We are a new creation because of what Jesus has done for us. Old things—old mentalities and ways of looking at the world—have passed away. Our mind has been changed. We do not see things or act the way we did before when our mind is renewed in Christ.

Being born again as a Christian does not necessarily mean that we already possess the mind of Christ. Instead, as Christians, we have the potential to receive the mind of Christ. As we all know, life holds many great battles and challenges. With a renewed mind, however, the Christian will not deal with problems the way that he or she did before coming to Christ. This is why we must be careful to guard our minds. Guarding our minds is essentially the same thing as what the Bible calls "being led by the Spirit." God will give us directions and insight into the world beyond our natural understanding or knowledge. The Holy Spirit will breathe life into the Word of God hidden in our hearts. But when we let the guard of our minds down, the enemy will penetrate our thoughts. As a result, we can have thoughts we never knew we were capable of having. These negative patterns of thought will ultimately bring despair and destruction.

Philippians 2:5 says, *"Let this mind be in you which was also in Christ Jesus."* When Paul says "let," he clearly means this is something we must allow to happen by the agreement of our wills. So what is the "mind of Christ"? The mind of Christ, first of all, is exemplified in the way Jesus submitted His will to the Heavenly Father. If we are to have the mind of Christ, we too must submit ourselves to God's plan. Dare we believe that it is possible to submit our minds to God in such a way that our thoughts become God's thoughts being expressed through us? Jesus understood that the Spirit of the Lord was upon Him, and the Spirit directed His ministry. Having the mind of Christ is being led by the Spirit.

We learn the mind of Christ by watching God's actions in Jesus. By observing His actions, we can back into His thoughts. For example, the Bible tells us that Jesus was moved by compassion for others. We see it in His actions. We see that there was no sickness so devastating that He could not heal it. There was no sin great enough that He could not forgive it. When we watch how Jesus handled the attacks of Satan, and how He handled suffering, we see that He never grew angry because of the difficulties He faced. To have the mind of Christ, then, we must watch Jesus closely—by seeing His actions we learn His thoughts.

Finally, in order to have the mind of Christ, we must have our priorities in order. He never lost sight of His focus. Nothing could take Jesus away from His mission, even the prospect of His own death. When Jesus went to the mountain after fasting for forty days, He was weak in the flesh. That's when Satan came to tempt Him. Don't be fooled; just like Jesus, the enemy will come to attack you when you are at your weakest point. After you have climbed your mountain, the devil will tempt you. When it looks like your friends have forsaken you and all is lost, Satan will oppose you. When the winds of adversity and doubt are blowing, the devil will come to offer you the kingdoms of this world and to plant thoughts in your mind that could eventually bring death to you. All he wants is for you to bow before him and compromise. When you get to this point, however, remember the mind we see demonstrated in Christ. Jesus, no doubt tired and weary, turned on his tormentor and said, "Satan, you get behind me!"

Learning to Sleep Through the Storm

When you have the mind of Christ, you will find peace in the middle of the storm. God wants you to be at peace, just as Jesus was when He slept through a great windstorm (Mark 4:35-41). He does not want you to be fearful but confident that He is watching over you. As the psalmist said in the midst of battle, *"I lay down and slept; I awoke, for the Lord sustained me"* (Psalm 3:5).

Our peace is not dependent on the storms that may swirl around us. Peace doesn't mean the storm is gone. Peace means learning how to be still and not fretful, confident and not anxious, even in the middle of the storm. That's the kind of peace Jesus gave us. He said, *"Peace I leave with you, My peace I give to you; not as the world gives do I give to you. Let not your heart be troubled, neither let it be afraid"* (John 14:27). Do not allow anxiety and fear to control your decisions. Though He was not immune to our struggles and trials, Jesus remained calm in the midst of adversity. We too can rejoice with the Psalmist if we have the mind of Christ:

"The Lord is my light and my salvation:
Whom shall I fear?
The Lord is the strength of my life;
Of whom shall I be afraid?
When the wicked came against me
To eat up my flesh, My enemies and foes,
They stumbled and fell.
Though an army should encamp against me,
In this I will be confident."
(Psalm 27:1-3)

Principles of Peace

1. *You have to know who you are in Christ.*
   Don't allow the devil to discourage you or to
   put false ideas in your mind about yourself
   and your purpose in life.

2. *Do not waver.* Stick to your destiny. Don't
   allow your negative attitudes and emotions
   to take you away from the original purpose
   for which you were born.

3. *Learn the art of casting your care on Him.*
   God wants to carry your burdens, so you
   don't have to.

4. *Learn how to bring your thoughts into captivity.* When we allow our thoughts to get
   away from us and plunge into negativity, we
   can affect our physical health.

5. *Begin and end your day with spiritual meditation.* Focusing on God will give you the
   peace necessary to handle the ups and downs
   of life.

6. *Take no thought for tomorrow.* We can live without anxiety because God is in control. Plain and simple: don't worry.

7. *Commit your total life to the glory of God.* Sometimes God will allow difficult situations. But our faith cannot help but glorify Him, even when we wrestle with pain we can't understand. Commit yourself to God, trusting that *"all things work together for good to those who love God and are the called according to His purpose"* (Romans 8:28).

I cannot tell you that you will ever reach the place where there are no battles. At the writing of this book, I am 74 years old. I became a Christian when I was a child. I have been preaching for 57 years. I have experienced the loss of parents, a sister, a daughter, and many of my natural family. I have endured my home burning and fought a battle with cancer. I can only tell you that my greatest desire has always been to finish the course that God has laid out for me.

I would like to end this book by assuring you that I have found God to be faithful. And I trust that as you have read this book that you have sensed my undying faith in a loving and compassionate Heavenly Father. My greatest legacy will be the seed that I have sown in the lives of young people that will follow me with an even greater faith and a more convincing word from God. I am praying for you.

PRAYERS

• • • • • • • • • • • • • • • • •

Lord, I know You are a good God. You want me to be well and strong. You sent Jesus Christ as the Great Physician. I stand today to declare, "You are my God!" I want to cooperate with You so that I can be well. Thank You for our physicians and their hospitals. Thank You for all the medicine you placed in the earth. Now I pray in the faith that I have in the Lord Jesus Christ. I thank You that I am being made whole of any infirmity I may have today. I am being made whole. I will think positively. I will speak positively. I will live in a community of love. I will love You, Father, with all that I have. I will love my neighbor even as I love myself. And now I give You praise, because I am well and whole, in the name of Jesus! Amen

• • • • • • • • • • • • • • • • •

How dare I as a man even have a thought that perhaps I might understand Your mind, Lord? And yet, when the question was asked, "Who can know the mind of the Lord," the Apostle responded, "But we have the mind of Christ." I pray today, Father, that You will take me to places I have never been. Let me hear sounds I have never heard. Let me think thoughts I have never thought. Let me experience You face-to-face. I am in Your hands Lord. In Jesus' name, I pray. Amen.

• • • • • • • • • • • • • • • • • • • •

Father, I pray not only for myself but for anyone I know who has need of healing. Let now Your Holy Spirit minister the power of healing that has been provided for us through the suffering of our Lord. By the Spirit of God, I come against the sickness or the disease that has invaded the life of this loved one. Let Your compassionate love be extended to our mortal bodies. Strengthen our minds so that we may overcome the power of unbelief. I now declare Your healing power present in our body to bring us to the well-being that You so desire for us to have. Let us now prosper and be in health even as our soul prospers, in Jesus' name. Amen.

Scriptures for
Self-Encouragement

All scripture references are given in the King James Version.

Exodus 23:25

And ye shall serve the LORD your God, and he shall bless thy bread, and thy water; and I w i l l take sickness away from the midst of thee.

Psalm 66:10

For thou, O God, hast proved us: thou hast tried us, as silver is tried.

Psalm 66:11

Thou broughtest us into the net; thou laidst affliction upon our loins.

Psalm 66:12

Thou hast caused men to ride over our heads; we went through fire and through water: but thou broughtest us out into a wealthy [place].

Psalm 84:11

For the LORD God [is] a sun and shield: the LORD will give grace and glory: no good [thing] will he withhold from them that walk uprightly.

Psalm 91:10

There shall no evil befall thee, neither shall any plague come nigh thy dwelling.

Psalm 103:1

Bless the LORD, O my soul: and all that is within me, [bless] his holy name.

Psalm 103:2

Bless the LORD, O my soul, and forget not all his benefits:

Psalm 103:3-5

Who forgiveth all thine iniquities; who healeth all thy diseases; Who redeemeth thy life from destruction; who crowneth thee with lovingkindness and tender mercies; Who satisfieth thy mouth with good [things; so that] thy youth is renewed like the eagle's.

Psalm 107:20
He sent his word, and healed them, and delivered [them] from their destructions.

Psalm 118:17
I shall not die, but live, and declare the works of the LORD.

Psalm 138:7
Though I walk in the midst of trouble, thou wilt revive me: thou shalt stretch forth thine hand against the wrath of mine enemies, and thy right hand shall save me.

Psalm 138:8
The LORD will perfect [that which] concerneth me: thy mercy, O LORD, endureth for ever: forsake not the works of thine own hands.

Proverbs 3:24

When thou liest down, thou shalt not be afraid: yea, thou shalt lie down, and thy sleep shall be sweet.

Proverbs 4:20

My son, attend to my words; incline thine ear unto my sayings.

Proverbs 4:21

Let them not depart from thine eyes; keep them in the midst of thine heart.

Proverbs 4:22

For they [are] life unto those that find them, and health to all their flesh.

Proverbs 4:23

Keep thy heart with all diligence; for out of it [are] the issues of life.

Isaiah 53:4

Surely he hath borne our griefs, and carried our sorrows: yet we did esteem him stricken, smitten of God, and afflicted.

Isaiah 53:5

But he [was] wounded for our transgressions, [he was] bruised for our iniquities: the chastisement of our peace [was] upon him; and with his stripes we are healed.

Jeremiah 30:17

For I will restore health unto thee, and I will heal thee of thy wounds, saith the LORD; because they called thee an Outcast, [saying], This [is] Zion, whom no man seeketh after.

Matthew 8:17

That it might be fulfilled which was spoken by Isaiah the prophet, saying, Himself took our infirmities, and bare [our] sicknesses.

Mark 11:24

Therefore I say unto you, What things soever ye desire, when ye pray, believe that ye receive [them], and ye shall have [them].

John 10:10

The thief cometh not, but for to steal, and to kill, and to destroy: I am come that they might have life, and that they might have [it] more abundantly.

John 11:4

When Jesus heard [that], he said, This sickness is not unto death, but for the glory of God, that the Son of God might be glorified thereby.

Romans 8:11

But if the Spirit of him that raised up Jesus from the dead dwell in you, he that raised up Christ from the dead shall also quicken your mortal bodies by his Spirit that dwelleth in you.

1 Corinthians 10:13

There hath no temptation taken you but such as is common to man: but God [is] faithful, who will not suffer you to be tempted above that ye are able; but will with the temptation also make a way to escape, that ye may be able to bear [it].

2 Corinthians 4:18

While we look not at the things which are seen, but at the things which are not seen: for the things which are seen [are] temporal; but the things which are not seen [are] eternal.

2 Corinthians 10:4-5

For the weapons of our warfare [are] not carnal, but mighty through God to the pulling down of strong holds; Casting down imaginations, and every high thing that exalteth itself against the knowledge of God, and bringing into captivity every thought to the obedience of Christ;

Philippians 4:13

I can do all things through Christ which strengtheneth me.

Hebrew 13:5

[Let your] conversation [be] without covetousness; [and be] content with such things as ye have: for he hath said, I will never leave thee, nor forsake thee.

James 5:1

Go to now, [ye] rich men, weep and howl for your miseries that shall come upon [you].

James 5:2

Your riches are corrupted, and your garments are motheaten.

James 5:3

Your gold and silver is cankered; and the rust of them shall be a witness against you, and shall eat your flesh as it were fire. Ye have heaped treasure together for the last days.

James 5:4

Behold, the hire of the labourers who have reaped down your fields, which is of you kept back by fraud, crieth: and the cries of them which have reaped are entered into the ears of the Lord of sabaoth.

James 5:5

Ye have lived in pleasure on the earth, and been wanton; ye have nourished your hearts, as in a day of slaughter.

James 5:6

Ye have condemned [and] killed the just; [and] he doth not resist you.

James 5:7

Be patient therefore, brethren, unto the coming of the Lord. Behold, the husbandman waiteth for the precious fruit of the earth, and hath long pa-

tience for it, until he receive the early and latter rain.

James 5:8

Be ye also patient; stablish your hearts: for the coming of the Lord draweth nigh.

James 5:9

Grudge not one against another, brethren, lest ye be condemned: behold, the judge standeth before the door.

James 5:10

Take, my brethren, the prophets, who have spoken in the name of the Lord, for an example of suffering affliction, and of patience.

James 5:11

Behold, we count them happy which endure. Ye have heard of the patience of Job, and have seen the end of the Lord; that the Lord is very pitiful, and of tender mercy.

James 5:12

But above all things, my brethren, swear not, neither by heaven, neither by the earth, neither by any other oath: but let your yea be yea; and [your] nay, nay; lest ye fall into condemnation.

James 5:13

Is any among you afflicted? let him pray. Is any merry? let him sing psalms.

James 5:14

Is any sick among you? let him call for the elders of the church; and let them pray over him, anointing him with oil in the name of the Lord:

James 5:15

And the prayer of faith shall save the sick, and the Lord shall raise him up; and if he have committed sins, they shall be forgiven him.

1 Peter 2:24

Who his own self bare our sins in his own body on the tree, that we, being dead to sins, should live unto righteousness: by whose stripes ye were healed.

1 John 3:21

*Beloved, if our heart condemn us not, [then] have
we confidence toward God.*

1 John 3:22

*And whatsoever we ask, we receive of him, be-
cause we keep his commandments, and do those
things that are pleasing in his sight.*

1 John 5:4

*For whatsoever is born of God overcometh the
world: and this is the victory that overcometh the
world, [even] our faith.*

1 John 5:14

*And this is the confidence that we have in him,
that, if we ask any thing according to his will, he
heareth us:*

1 John 5:15

*And if we know that he hear us, whatsoever we
ask, we know that we have the petitions that we
desired of him.*

Jude 1:20

But ye, beloved, building up yourselves on your most holy faith, praying in the Holy Spirit,

Jude 1:21

Keep yourselves in the love of God, looking for the mercy of our Lord Jesus Christ unto eternal life.

Revelation 12:11

And they overcame him by the blood of the Lamb, and by the word of their testimony; and they loved not their lives unto the death.

Songs in the Night

Lord I Hope this Day is Good

Words & Music by Dave Hanner
Published by Sabal Music Inc. (ASCAP)

Lord I hope this day is good
I'm feeling empty like you know I would
I should be thankful, Lord, I know I should
But Lord I hope this day is good
Lord, have you forgotten me
I've been praying to you faithfully
I'm not saying I am a righteous man
Lord I know you understand
I don't need fortune and I don't need fame
Send down the thunder, send down the rain
But when you are planning just how it will be
Plan a good day for me

(Chorus)
You've been the King since the dawn of time
All that I'm asking is a less cry
It might be hard for the devil to do
But it would be easy for you.

Whispering Hope
Published by Alice Hawthorne

Soft as the voice of an Angel,
Breathing a lesson unheard,
Hope with a gentle persuasion
Whispers her comforting word.
Wait, till the darkness is over,
Wait, till the tempest is done,
Hope for the sunshine tomorrow
After the shower is gone.

Refrain:
|: Whispering hope,
  Oh, how welcome thy voice,
  Making my heart
  In its sorrow rejoice. :|

Hope has an anchor so steadfast,
Rends the dark veil for the soul.
Whither the Master has entered,
Robbing the grave of its goal.
Come then O come glad fruition,
Come to my sad weary heart.
Come Thou O blessed hope of glory,
Never O never depart.

Refrain:

If in the dusk of the twilight,
Dim be the region afar,
Will not the deepening darkness
Brighten the glimmering star?
Then, when the night is upon us,
Why should the heart sink away?
When the dark midnight is over
Watch for the breaking of day.
Refrain:

Trading My Sorrows (Yes Lord)
Published by Darrell Evans

I am trading my sorrows
I am trading my shame.
I am laying them down for the joy of the Lord.
I am trading my sickness. I am trading my pain.
I am laying them down for the joy of the Lord
Yes Lord, yes Lord, yes, yes Lord.
Yes Lord, yes Lord, yes, yes Lord.
Yes Lord, yes Lord, yes, yes Lord amen.
I am pressed but not crushed,
Persecuted not abandoned,
Struck down but not destroyed.
I am blessed beyond the curse for
His promise will endure,
That his joy's gonna be my strength,
Though the sorrow may last for the night,
Joy comes with the morning.

1998 Integrity's Hosanna! Music (ASCAP)

Prophecy for Healing

Prophecy to Bishop Earl Paulk by
Pastor Tommy Reid on
October 1, 2000:

*"As much as you have preached that the King-
dom of God is now present, you have yet to know
the true power of the Kingdom. You are about to
move into the NOW. You have been well acquainted with the God of the past. No one can
preach that like the Bishop. You have heard the
stories. You've heard them declared as relevant
to the present. You have believed for the actions
of God for the future: 'I will be healed.' God will
take this church into its divine destiny—the God
of the future. But you are prophetically about to
become acquainted with the God of the NOW in
the NOW. I have a word for this church. "You
are about to enter the NOW of the prophetic voice.
This is the day when God is about to release the*

prophetic voice of this Bishop. The devil has attempted to silence it. Here is the word of God to you: the day of silence is over and the day at this age in your life has come when the world will hear the voice of the prophet. Secondly, you are about to move into the NOW of your witness and your influence upon culture. That day has come. The salt of your witness has gradually come out of its shaker and the salt of that witness is about to be tasted by the world. The witness of this house shall be seen by the world as it gradually begins to infiltrate the cultures of our day.

"And then the Lord has a specific prophetic word for you Bishop, I believe, based on the covenant promise in III John 2: 'Beloved, I wish above all things that you may prosper, that you may be in health (you need that today) just as your soul prospers.' You, this house and this Bishop, are about to enter the NOW fulfillment of that covenant promise

"First, regarding money: Today, you took a Harvester offering --- a double tithe. You in this house shall see the demonstration of God's prosperity of the Abrahamic covenant. God's prosperity shall come to pass even to the complete eradication of *the debt on this building. God's going to miraculously provide for that. Your health, Bishop: as much as you have suffered, you shall NOW begin to live in the divine health personally guaranteed by this covenant. You have always believed it. For the days of your pain and your weakness have come to an end because of the realization and the activation of the covenant you have always preached. I declare to you right now that the weakness you see in your body shall not plague you this week. It's your beginning of a new life.*

"Here is a word God has specifically given me and I have never seen this before, and I've never heard anyone say this before, but God so breathed into my spirit that I have to tell it to you. Your soul: your emotions, your mind, and your will shall know prosperity! Because it says 'as your soul prospers.' Let me tell you what I think this means. Your mind shall know that Covenant. Your mind is going to be filled with the greatest creative ideas that you have ever had --- far beyond the creative ideas of your youth. Your mind shall know that covenant. Your mind will be filled with creative ideas that you have never heard before or seen before. Many times we look at those

of us who are older and wonder if we can be as creative as we were back in our past, but God is going to activate the covenant of your mind -the prosperity of your mind.

"Secondly, your emotions will experience a meaningful change. You've always been a man who decided in the midst of all the problems to be happy --- to be an overcomer. You decided to be full of joy even when there was no reason for it. But your emotions are about to enter a new dimension. All your tears are going to be turned into God's joy.

"Lastly, (this is so in my spirit and I don't know how to say it or write it adequately) you have always willed --- you've always been a man of determination, as long as I have known you. You have always willed to do God's will. However, for the first time in your life, your will shall not be in your own strength. You have always set yourself like a flint to do God's will. But your will shall literally be inspired by God. A 'God determination' will come into your spirit. It will set itself like a flint: number one, to live long, and number two, your will shall be set to the absolute

fulfillment of God's dreams and goals for your life. For you, Bishop, and this house, are about to enter the NOW of God."

A Testimony

A Testimony sent from Beverly Vanessa Martin, staff member of Cathedral of the Holy Spirit

As recommended, I scheduled a routine mammogram in October of 1999. Going into the office that day, I had no idea that this procedure was going to end up as anything but another "routine" visit. The mammogram results came back normal, as usual, except for a small shadow. The technicians and doctors agreed that this finding needed further investigation. This, of course, involved an actual biopsy. Then the final report came back that this ambiguous shadow was indeed a cancerous situation. I just could not believe this was happening to me, certainly not. I cried and then cried some more. Finally, I cried out to God. And He heard me, as He always does. And I felt His presence in a new and special way.

I was ready for the battle. This cancer may have made itself welcome as an uninvited guest, but I determined that it was not going to be in control any longer. I surrounded myself with those who would be a help and encouragement. My husband, Hal, was so vital throughout this entire process. He made sure we were properly submitted to the eldership of our church for prayer and counsel. Most of all, Hal had a way of knowing when to let me cry and then when to dry the tears and send me out to face another day. I truly had a wonderful support system in my friends and family, but there were still many times where it was just the Lord and me. Upon a suggestion from a friend, I wrote key Scriptures down on index cards. If I began to feel down, I would pull these out and read them until I was ready to move forward again. Having done all, I simply (and often not so simply) stood firm and let God do the rest.

And He never disappointed me. He was with me all the way. The medical personnel marveled at my condition—both physically and emotionally. At every juncture, the doctors would outline what I should expect to happen. And every time, I refused to accept anything that would interfere with my work for the Kingdom of God. With His help and grace, I did not miss one day of work or one Sunday of ushering. It was a constant battle, but I was going to show the enemy what I was capable of doing. In fact, the Lord made sure I never had a moment to sit around and mope, because I always had something coming up.

After being cut, poisoned, and burned, I have to say that I don't know if life will ever be "as usual" again. But, I can say that for this too I am grateful. I will never be satisfied with life as usual again. I will never see life as usual. It is truly unusual—with blessings in many different shapes and forms all along the way.

Whom You Should Contact

National Cancer Institute
1-800-4-CANCER
1-800-422-6237
wwwicic.nci.nih.gov

American Cancer Society
National Office
1599 Clifton Road N.E.
Atlanta, GA 30329
1-800-ACS-2345
1-800-227-2345
www.cancer.org

Division Offices

Alabama

504 Brookwood Blvd.
Homewood, AL 35209
205-879-2242

Alaska
1057 West Fireweed Lane
Anchorage, AK 99503
907-277-8696

Arizona
2929 East Thomas Road
Phoenix, AZ 85016
602-224-0524

Arkansas
901 North University
Little Rock, AR 72203
501-644-3480

California
1720 Webster Street
Oakland, CA 96412
510-893-7900

Colorado
2255 South Oneida
Denver, CO 80224
303-758-2030

Connecticut
Barns Park South
14 Village Lane
Wallingtford, CT 06492
203-265-7161

Delaware
92 Read's Way
Suite 205
New Castle, DE 19720
302-324-4227

District of Columbia
1875 Connecticut Avenue, N.W.
Suite 730
Washington, DC 20009
202-483-2600

Florida
3709 West Jetton Avenue
Tampa, FL 33629-5146
813-253-0541

Georgia
2200 Lake Boulevard
Atlanta, GA 30319
404-816-7800

Hawaii
Community Service Center Building
200 North Vineyard Blvd.
Suite 100A
Honolulu, HI 96817

Idaho
2676 Vista Avenue
Boise, ID 83705-0386
208-343-4609

Illinois
77 East Monroe
Chicago, IL 60603-5795
312-641-6150

Indiana
8730 Commerce Park Place
Indianapolis, IN 46268
317-872-4432

Iowa

8364 Hickman Rd.

Des Moines, IA 50325

515-253-0147

Kansas

1315 S.W. Arrowhead Rd.

Topeka, KS 66604

913-273-4114

Kentucky

701 West Muhammad Ali Blvd.

Louisville, KY 40201-1807

502-584-6782

Louisiana

2200 Veteran's Memorial Blvd.

Kenner, LA 70062

504-469-0021

Maine

52 Federal St.

Brunswick, ME 040011

207-729-3339

Maryland
8219 Town Circle Dr.
Baltimore, MD 21236-0026
410-931-6850

Massachusetts
30 Speen St.
Framingham, MA 01701-9376
508-270-4600

Michigan
1205 East Saginaw St.
Lansing, MI 48906
517-371-2920

Minnesota
3316 West 66th St.
Minneapolis, MN 55435
612-925-2772

Mississippi
1380 Livingston Ln.
Lakeover Office Park
Jackson, MI 39213
601-362-8874

Missouri
3322 American Ave.
Jefferson City, MO 65102
314-893-4800

Montana
17 North 26th St.
Billings, MT 59101
406-252-7111

Nebraska
8502 West Center Rd.
Omaha, NE 68124-5255
402-393-5800

Nevada
1325 East Harmon
Las Vegas, NV 89119
702-798-6857

New Hampshire
360 Route 101, Unit 501
Bedford, NH 03110-5032
603-472-8899

New Jersey
2600 US Highway 1
North Brunswick, NJ 08902-0803
908-297-8000

New Mexico
5800 Lomas Boulevard, NE
Albuquerque, NM 87110
505-260-2105

New York State
6725 Lyons St.
East Syracuse, NY 13057
315-437-7025

Long Island
75 Davids Dr.
Hauppauge, NY 11788
516-436-7070

New York City
19 West 56th St.
New York, NY 10019
212-586-8700

Queens

112-25 Queens Blvd.

Forest Hill, NY 11375

718-263-2224

Westchester

2 Lyon Place

White Plains, NY 10601

914-949-4800

North Carolina

11 South Boylan Ave.

Raleigh, NC 27603

919-834-8463

North Dakota

123 Roberts St.

Fargo, ND 58102

701-231-1385

Ohio

5555 Frantz Rd.

Dublin, OH 43017

614-889-9565

Oklahoma
4323 63rd, Suite 110
Oklahoma City, OK 73116
405-843-9888

Oregon
0330 S.W. Curry
Portland, OR 97201
503-295-6422

Pennsylvania
Route 422 & Sipe Avenue
Hershey, PA 17033-0897
717-533-6144

Philadelphia
1422 Chestnut St.
Philadelphia, PA 19102
215-665-2900

Puerto Rico
Calle Alverio No.577
Esquina Sargento Medina
Hato Rey, PR 00918
809-764-2295

Rhode Island
400 Main Street
Pawtucket, RI 02860
401-722-8480

South Carolina
128 Stonemark Lane
Columbia, SC 29210-3855
803-750-1693

South Dakota
4101 Carnegie Place
Sioux Falls, SD 57106-2322
605-361-8977

Tennessee
1315 Eighth Avenue,
South Nashville, TN 37203
615-255-1227

Texas
2433 Ridgepoint Drive
Austin, TX 75356
512-928-2262

Utah
941 East 3300 South
Salt Lake City, UT 84106
801-4831500

Vermont
13 Loomis St.
Montpelier, VT 05602
802-223-2348

Virginia
4240 Park Place Court
Glen Allen, VA 23060
804-527-3700

Washington
2120 First Avenue,
North Seattle,WA 98109-1140
206-283-1152

West Virginia
2428 Kanawha Boulevard
East Charleston, WV 25311
304-344-3611

Wisconsin
N19 W24350 Riverwood Drive
Waukesha, WI 53188
414-523-5500

Wyoming
4202 Ridge Rd.
Cheyenne, WY 82001
307-638-3331